Focus on Cocaine
and Crack

Focus on Cocaine and Crack
A Drug-Alert Book

Jeffrey Shulman
Illustrated by David Neuhaus

TWENTY-FIRST CENTURY BOOKS
FREDERICK, MARYLAND

Published by
Twenty-First Century Books
38 South Market Street
Frederick, Maryland 21701

Text Copyright © 1990
Twenty-First Century Books

Illustrations Copyright © 1990
David Neuhaus

Printed in the United States of America

10 9 8 7 6 5 4 3 2 1

Library of Congress Cataloging in Publication Data

Shulman, Jeffrey
Focus on Cocaine and Crack
Illustrated by David Neuhaus

(A Drug-Alert Book)
Includes bibliographical references.
Summary: Discusses how cocaine and crack affect the mind
and body and presents a brief history of cocaine use.
1. Cocaine—Juvenile literature.
2. Cocaine habit—United States—Juvenile literature.
[1. Cocaine. 2. Crack (Drug). 3. Drug Abuse.]
I. Neuhaus, David, ill. II. Title.
III. Series: The Drug-Alert Series.
HV5810.S58   1990
362.2'98'0973—dc20   89-20446 CIP AC
ISBN 0-941477-98-3

14.99

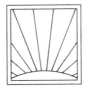

Table of Contents

Introduction

"Baby Saved by Miracle Drug!" "Drug Bust at Local School!" Headlines like these are often side by side in your newspaper, or you may hear them on the evening news. This is confusing. If drugs save lives, why are people arrested for having and selling them?

The word "drug" is part of the confusion. It is a word with many meanings. The drug that saves a baby's life is also called a medicine. The illegal drugs found at the local school have many names—names like pot, speed, and crack. But one name for all of these illegal drugs is dope.

Some medicines you can buy at your local drugstore or grocery store, and there are other medicines only a doctor can get for you. But whether you buy them yourself or need a doctor to order them for you, medicines are made to get you healthy when you are sick.

Dope is not for sale in any store. You can't get it from a doctor. Dope is bought from someone called a "dealer" or a "pusher" because using, buying, or selling dope is against the law. That doesn't stop some people from using dope. They say they do it to change the way they feel. Often, that means they are trying to run away from their problems. But when the dope wears off, the problems are still there—and they are often worse than before.

There are three drugs we see so often that we sometimes forget they really are drugs. These are alcohol, nicotine, and caffeine. Alcohol is in beer, wine, and liquor. Nicotine is found in cigarettes, cigars, pipe tobacco, and other tobacco products. Caffeine is in coffee, tea, soft drinks, and chocolate. These three drugs are legal. They are sold in stores. But that doesn't mean they are always safe to use. Alcohol and nicotine are such strong drugs that only adults are allowed to buy and use them. And most parents try to keep their children from having too much caffeine.

Marijuana, cocaine, alcohol, nicotine, caffeine, medicines: these are all drugs. All drugs are alike because they change the way our bodies and minds work. But different drugs cause different changes. Some help, and some harm. And when they aren't used properly, even helpful drugs can harm us.

Figuring all this out is not easy. That's why The Drug-Alert Books were written: so you will know why certain drugs are used, how they affect people, why they are dangerous, and what laws there are to control them.

Knowing about drugs is important. It is important to you and to all the people who care about you.

David Friedman, Ph.D.
Consulting Editor

Dr. David Friedman is Deputy Director of the Division of Preclinical Research at the National Institute on Drug Abuse.

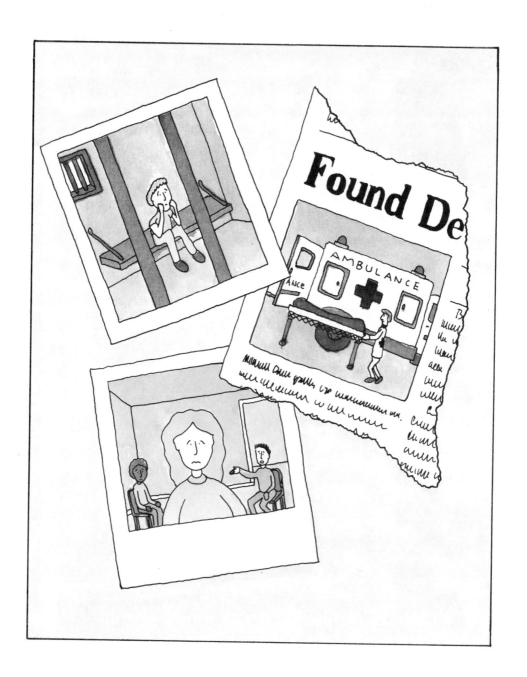

The Cocaine Picture

A young girl sits in a drug treatment center in New York City. She is hooked on crack. "It took over me," she says. "It was like a monster took over my body and mind."

The 14-year-old boy is a messenger in the Washington, D.C., cocaine trade. He is sitting behind bars. In the early hours of a hot August morning, he shot and killed two men. A police officer explains that "he was a young boy trying to look big, trying to be a soldier in the drug war."

The phone call to the emergency room comes too late. By the time the ambulance gets to the dormitory, the star college basketball player is dead. Cocaine killed him.

These are pictures of people who used cocaine and crack. They are different pictures, but they all tell the same story.

You have probably heard about cocaine. You may have read reports of famous movie stars or athletes who got in trouble with cocaine. You may have seen news stories about the violent world of cocaine dealers, smugglers, and users. It's not surprising that cocaine is so much in the news. In the last 20 years, more and more people have tried cocaine—over 22 million Americans. Today, over 5 million people use it each month. Each day, 3,000 people try cocaine for the first time.

You probably have questions about cocaine.

- What is this drug?

- Why do so many people use it?

- Why, if it is so dangerous, do people use it at all?

- Why do they continue to use it even when they know how harmful it is?

- Why do I need to know about it?

Cocaine is a drug that changes the way the brain works. It changes the way people think, feel, and behave. One reason why cocaine is now used so much is that people don't know the facts about it. They think using it is fun and glamorous. They may think that it is safer than other drugs. They think that they won't get addicted to it.

But they are wrong. Scientists and doctors believe that cocaine is one of the most dangerous of all drugs. Dr. Mark S. Gold, the director of the National Cocaine Hotline, says, "Callers to our help line tell us that they cannot stop using cocaine even though they know it is destroying their lives."

It is important for everyone to know the truth about cocaine. It is especially important for you and your friends to know about cocaine because young people are now using it. Cocaine is not just a problem for adults. It's a problem for young people, too. One in every 10 teenagers tries cocaine. One high-school counselor was recently asked to describe cocaine use among school-age children today: "Younger and younger, and more and more" was his report.

It is important for you to know about cocaine because some young people are now using crack, one of the most dangerous forms of cocaine. Today, the average age of a crack user is only 17 years old.

If this book had been written in 1985, it would not have mentioned crack. No one had heard of it yet.

Dr. Gold founded 800-COCAINE, a national hotline to help people with cocaine problems, in 1983. By mid 1985 the hotline had received more than a million calls. Not one of those calls mentioned crack. One year later, nearly one-half of all the people who called 800-COCAINE wanted to talk about the new form of cocaine called crack.

Who are these cocaine and crack users?

- They are people like Leslie, just 13 years old. When she was 12, Leslie was living on the streets and spending $200 a day on cocaine.

- They are people like Don Rogers, a star football player for the Cleveland Browns. He used cocaine at a party only two days before he was going to be married. He died the next morning.

- They are people like Monica. She is now in a drug-treatment program for cocaine use. She was caught stealing money from her parents to buy crack. "I never thought this would happen to me," she said.

These are pictures of a drug that is destroying thousands of lives every day. Cocaine is a drug that hurts the rich and the poor, the young and the old. It is a drug that tears apart the life of small towns and big cities. Cocaine users are found in every job and in every walk of life. It is a drug that affects us all.

Different pictures, but they all tell the same story.

What Is Cocaine?

Cocaine is a white powder made from the leaves of the coca plant. Cocaine is taken from the coca leaf in two steps. First, the leaves are pressed to form a coca paste; then, the paste is treated with very strong chemicals to make a white, powdery mixture. Cocaine looks like powdered sugar or baby powder. The kind of cocaine known as crack is made from cocaine powder. Crack comes in small chips or "rocks" that look like little pieces of soap.

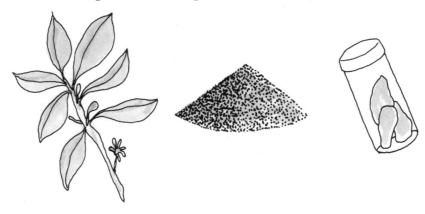

Cocaine has many names. "Coke," "snow," "toot," "C," "blow," "nose candy," and "The Lady" are just some of them. But whatever you call it, cocaine is a dangerous drug. It can even be deadly.

People who use cocaine say a dose or "hit" of coke gives them a burst or "rush" of excitement. They say they have more energy when they use it. They get a feeling of power.

This is how some people describe being high on cocaine:

"I was filled with an incredible feeling. I felt beautiful and important, on the top of my world."

"After one hit of cocaine, I felt like a new man."

"It made my body say, 'I want more. I want some more.'"

People who use cocaine don't really care what causes this feeling of energy and power. But if they knew why cocaine makes them feel this way, they would think twice about using such a dangerous drug.

Cocaine is a kind of drug called a stimulant. That means it speeds up the way the brain works. You can imagine what that feels like.

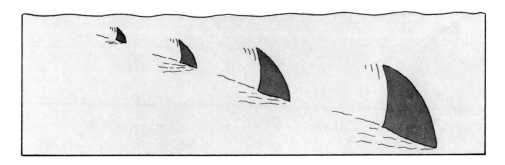

Imagine you are sitting in a dark theater. The movie is about a monstrous shark who attacks without warning. Then, suddenly, you see the dark fin of the deadly monster. Silently and quickly, the shark is moving closer and closer to the people on the beach . . . closer and closer. . . . You want to shout out . . . you clutch the arms of your seat . . . your heart feels like it will burst out of your chest, . . . and, then, just as suddenly, a boy with a shark-fin inner tube pops up out of the water and shouts, "Surprise!" You breathe an immense sigh of relief—"Phew!"—and feel your body begin to relax.

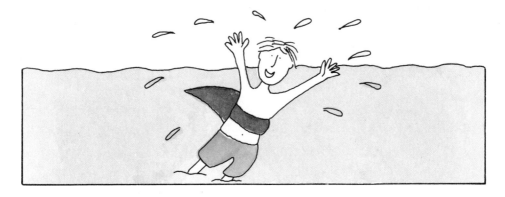

Or, remember what it feels like to be on a roller coaster ride, climbing slowly . . . slowly . . . to the top. Your heart is beating fast, you're breathing hard, your mind is racing, and your whole body feels on edge.

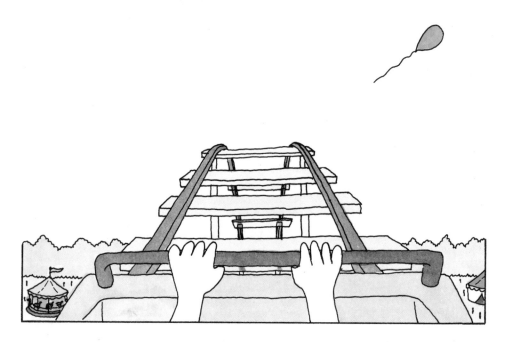

This is how your body responds to danger, whether the danger is real or imaginary. It is called the "fight or flight" response. When you seem to be in danger, your brain sends out special chemicals that get your body ready to fight or run away. You can't control the fight or flight response. But you can make the response happen.

You make the fight or flight response happen when you put yourself in danger. That's what you do when you watch a scary movie or when you ride a roller coaster. Your brain gets your body ready to fight or run away, even if the danger is only a movie or an amusement park ride.

Why do you like to watch scary movies? Why do you like to ride the roller coaster? Have you ever thought, "Why do I do this to myself?"

You do it because it's fun. You like the feeling of excitement. You like the feeling of energy. You like the stimulation.

Cocaine also causes the fight or flight response to happen. When a person uses cocaine, the brain and body release the same kind of chemicals that help people respond to danger. The heart and lungs work faster. There is the same feeling of excitement and stimulation. When a person uses cocaine, the brain gets the body ready to fight or run away, even though there is no real danger.

Cocaine also increases the amount of the chemicals in the brain that cause feelings of pleasure and self-confidence. The brain controls our feelings and moods. Chemicals in the brain can make us feel happy or upset, angry or calm. Cocaine produces a feeling of wellness, the kind of feeling that says, "There's nothing I can't do." This feeling is often called "euphoria." It means a feeling of great happiness. People use cocaine, again and again, to get this feeling.

But this feeling is not true happiness. It is just the coke high, and it doesn't last long. When it wears off, the cocaine user often feels terrible. Sad, nervous, irritable, confused, angry, tired—this is how cocaine users feel when they are no longer high. This feeling is called a cocaine "crash."

The effects of cocaine may last from 5 to 40 minutes. How long the effects last depends on the way a person uses cocaine. There are three different ways of taking cocaine.

The way people use cocaine most often is by sniffing the cocaine powder through the nose. When cocaine is sniffed, it enters the bloodstream through the small blood vessels of the nose. The bloodstream carries the cocaine throughout the body. It takes about 10 to 15 minutes for the effects of cocaine to start. They last about 30 to 40 minutes.

Some people give themselves shots of cocaine. They inject a mixture of cocaine and water into the body by using a hypodermic needle. Used this way, the drug goes straight into the body's bloodstream. Injecting cocaine gets a person high in about 15 seconds. The effects usually last from 20 to 30 minutes.

Other people smoke cocaine by sprinkling the powder on a marijuana cigarette (called a joint). Still others smoke crack in special pipes. Smoking cocaine and crack also gets a person high right away. The effects last only 10 to 20 minutes.

People use cocaine to feel different. When they crash and start to feel bad, they often use coke again. "You had to get more," one teenage girl said, describing how she got started with cocaine. "You had to get more and more." It is the start of a cocaine problem.

How does a cocaine problem develop? Why do so many people who use it once end up using it again and again?

People learn to use coke just as they learn to do so many other things. One way you learn is by being rewarded when you do something well. A reward makes you feel good. When you get a reward for doing something well, you want to do it again. The effects of using cocaine are like that. When people use cocaine, the feeling of energy and power they get is like a reward. So people want to use cocaine again and again.

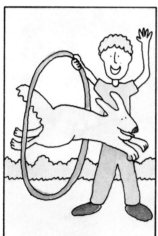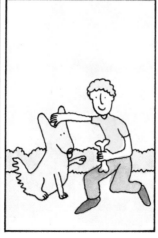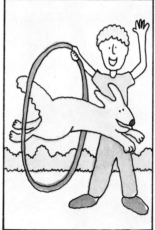

Cocaine may make people feel different for a little while, but using cocaine is a way of not facing up to life. Instead of solving problems, coke users turn to a drug to try to forget their problems. They may never try to face problems or feel good without cocaine. They are beginning to need the drug to be happy.

And, soon, they will need more and more of it. Scientists now know that coke users develop a tolerance to the drug. Tolerance means users need more and more of a drug to feel the same way they felt when they first started using it.

Using cocaine changes the brain so that coke users need another dose of the drug to feel normal. Their bodies need the cocaine, just like your body needs food or drink. This is called physical dependence. Their minds crave the drug: they feel they "must have" cocaine. This is called addiction.

Coke addicts may want to stop, but they are hooked. They need to get more and more of the drug. The coke habit is like a maze with no escape: the more people use coke, the more they need it; and the more they need it, the more they use it.

Imagine a scary movie that never ends. It just keeps getting scarier. Imagine a roller coaster ride that never stops. It just keeps getting faster. Imagine a nightmare from which you can't wake up. That's what being hooked on coke is like. Only worse, much worse.

You can't imagine how bad it is.

Crack

It seemed to come out of nowhere. Now, it seems to be everywhere.

It is found on the tough streets of big cities and in the quiet, tree-lined neighborhoods of the suburbs. You can buy it on 107th Street in New York City; you can buy it in small towns in Georgia.

A recent report said "the craze is spreading nationwide." Every day there are stories about it in the news. Every day people are arrested for selling and using it.

It is one of the most addictive drugs known.

It is crack.

Crack is cocaine that is made to be smoked. It is called crack because it makes a crackling sound when it is smoked. Because crack is smoked, it goes to work fast. It takes less than 10 seconds for crack to reach the brain.

Crack is a special problem for young people. There are many reasons why crack is being used by some young people:

- Crack can now be bought cheaply. A vial with two doses costs only about $10. But because crack users smoke so much of the drug, they end up spending as much money or more than other cocaine users.

- Crack is easy to find. Police officers in Los Angeles, Houston, Boston, Atlanta, Chicago, Baltimore, Washington, D.C., and dozens of other cities say the same thing: "It's everywhere."

- Some young people use crack because their friends are using it, too. They think that crack is the "in" drug to do.

- Crack is easy to use. Smoking crack in a pipe is easier than snorting cocaine powder, and many people don't like the idea of using needles to get the effects of cocaine.

- Some young people like the thrill of trying such a dangerous drug. Smoking crack gets a much bigger and stronger—and much more dangerous—dose of cocaine to the brain.

The effects of crack last from 5 to 20 minutes. Crack users say the effects are very powerful—a "super" high. Then comes the crash—and it is a bad one. The crash from using crack is much worse than the crash from sniffing cocaine powder. Some crack users say they feel like they are being "crushed." It is a super low.

Because the crack high lasts for such a short time and the crack low is so low, crack users take the drug again and again. That's why using crack is the easiest and quickest way to get addicted to cocaine. Medical experts say you can get hooked on crack in two weeks. But many users say they were hooked from the first time they tried it. One expert on drug use calls crack a "chance for instant addiction."

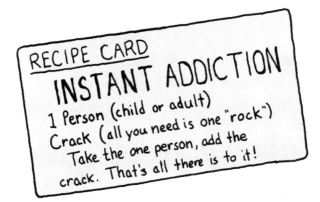

RECIPE CARD
INSTANT ADDICTION
1 Person (child or adult)
Crack (all you need is one "rock")
Take the one person, add the crack. That's all there is to it!

Crack is the newest part of the cocaine story. But the story of cocaine is an old one. It begins thousands of years ago.

The History of Cocaine

"The life of the people was a very harsh one. The air on the cold mountaintops was difficult to breathe, and the land was hard to farm. The people were often hungry and tired. The sun god Inti took pity on the Inca people. He asked his mother, the moon goddess Moma Quilla, to help the people in their distress. The great moon goddess smiled and sent her blessing to the Incas. It was a tall, sturdy bush—one that would live 50 years or more, one that would produce a strange power for the weary people of the mountains. It was the coca plant."

There are many folktales like this one about the coca plant. They tell of the great gift of the coca leaf.

The cocaine story is an old one—over 3,000 years old. It begins high in the mountain valleys of South America. There, on the steep slopes of the Andes Mountains, the coca plant grows wild.

Cocaine comes from the greenish-brown leaves of the coca plant. The Indians of South America have known for thousands of years that the leaves of the coca plant have a strange and stimulating power.

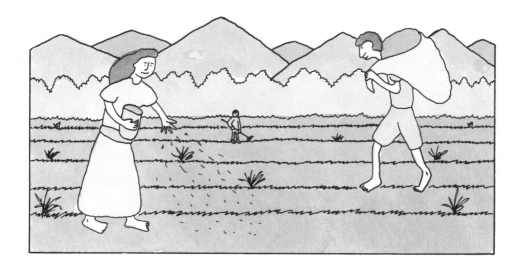

When the Indians chewed the leaves of the coca plant, they felt a surge of strength and energy. They were able to work harder and longer. They were able to work without rest. The coca leaves helped to deaden the pain of hunger and fatigue. In the harsh valleys of the Andes Mountains, it is hard work to make a living off the land. The power of the coca leaves seemed to be a blessing. The Indians of South America even thought the coca leaf was a gift from the gods.

What was the secret power of the coca leaves?

The surge of strength and energy felt by the Indians of the Andes did not come from the gods. It came from the active ingredient in the coca leaf. It was cocaine.

The Incas were conquered by soldiers from Spain in the 16th century. Such Spanish explorers as Francisco Pizarro came to the "New World" in search of great wealth. They heard of cities made of gold in the mountains of South America. Spanish soldiers conquered the Indian peoples and put them to work as slaves in the gold and silver mines of the Andes Mountains.

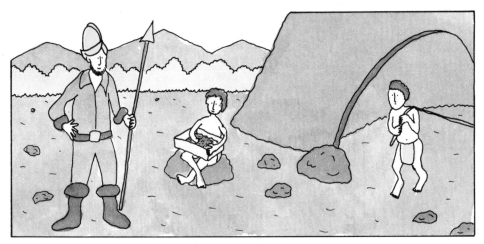

At first, the Spanish tried to stop the Indians from using the coca leaf. They wanted the Incas to become Christians, and they did not want the Indians to worship the "false god" of the coca leaf.

But the Spanish conquerors soon changed their minds about the coca plant. Gold and silver were more important to them than teaching the Indians to be Christians. The Spanish saw that the coca leaves gave the Indians energy to work long hours in the mines with little food or sleep. So the Spanish gave their Indian slaves coca leaves as a reward for their hard work. But this reward only made the Indians slaves to the cocaine habit, too.

Coca leaves were soon brought back to Europe from South America, but it was not until the mid 1800s that cocaine became popular there. In 1859, Albert Niemann was able to produce the white powder that held the secret power of the coca leaf. It was soon afterwards that scientists and doctors began to experiment with cocaine. They wanted to see if this new drug could be a useful medicine.

The most important of these scientists was a man named Sigmund Freud. Freud is most famous today for his work in treating mental illness. But in 1884, his research led him to study the effects of cocaine. Freud tried the drug on himself and other doctors, and he soon believed that cocaine was a miracle drug. He thought cocaine could relieve nervousness and depression, cure stomach problems and asthma, and ease pain. He even thought cocaine could be given as a cure for drug and alcohol abuse. It was only years later that Freud learned that cocaine is a harmful and addictive drug.

In part because of Freud's work, cocaine became a very popular drug in the late 1880s. It was used as an anesthetic, a drug that helps to relieve pain. Cocaine is still used as an anesthetic today in some special operations. But in the 1890s, it was also used as a general "cure-all" for problems like upset stomachs, allergies, and tiredness.

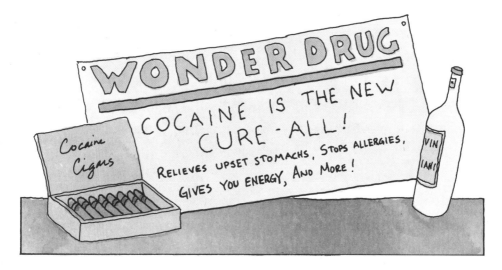

Several companies added cocaine to their products: there were cocaine cigars, teas, candies, and drinks. One cocaine drink was Vin Mariani. It was a mixture of cocaine and wine. Its inventor, Angelo Mariani, claimed that his new tonic was "unequaled for the overworked Body and Brain." Vin Mariani was widely used and was praised by such famous people as President Ulysses S. Grant, the inventor Thomas Edison, the writer Jules Verne, and Pope Leo XIII.

Coca-Cola

It may surprise you to learn that Coca-Cola used to contain cocaine.

In 1886, an American pharmacist made a new drink with cocaine as an ingredient. He called it "Coca-Cola." When Americans were feeling tired, they didn't have to go to the mountains of South America for a stimulant. Cocaine was as close by as the nearest soft drink.

"Tired?" asked an advertisement. "Then, drink Coca-Cola. It relieves exhaustion. When your brain is running under full pressure, send for a glass of Coca-Cola. You will be surprised how quickly it will ease the tired brain and soothe the rattled nerves."

In 1903, the Coca-Cola Company took the cocaine out of its drink. But the new Coca-Cola still contained caffeine, another stimulant.

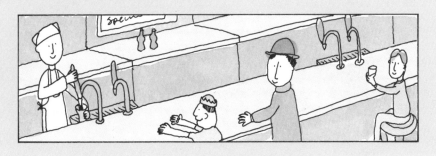

By 1900, it was clear that cocaine was not a miracle drug. People who used cocaine got hooked on it. Sigmund Freud reported that there were harmful side effects to cocaine use. Newspapers and magazines told stories of young men and women driven insane by cocaine addiction. And many doctors complained that cocaine products were dangerous.

Cocaine became less and less popular in the early 1900s. Doctors found safer drugs to ease pain, and companies began to take the cocaine out of their products. Laws were passed to control and restrict cocaine use. In the United States, the Harrison Narcotics Act of 1914 made the personal use of cocaine illegal and limited other uses of the drug. By the 1920s, cocaine was an almost forgotten drug.

But it was not totally forgotten. Cocaine became popular again in the 1970s. Many people thought coke was safer to use than other illegal drugs. In popular movies, glamorous people were seen using coke, and some famous music groups sang about cocaine. It was not long before cocaine became the "in" drug for people who lived life "in the fast lane"—from artists to lawyers, from rock stars to athletes.

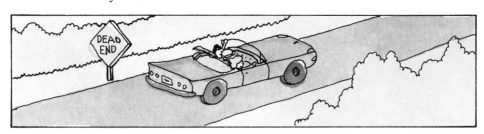

Cocaine was so expensive in the 1970s that only very rich people could afford to use it. But the more popular cocaine became, the cheaper it got. In the 1980s, the price of cocaine was low enough that most people, even high-school students, could afford to try it. The number of people who had used cocaine in 1974 was over 5 million; in 1982, the number was over 21 million.

The 1980s also saw new and more dangerous ways of using cocaine, such as mixing it with other drugs like heroin and PCP. Then, in 1986, there were the first reports of a new form of cocaine called crack.

Using, buying, or selling cocaine and crack is against the law. The laws vary from state to state, but in each state getting caught with cocaine is a serious crime. It can mean going to jail and paying a heavy fine.

Despite new, tougher laws, crack is now the "in" way to use cocaine for some young people. It is now the biggest drug problem in many cities. On almost any day, there is news of more violence related to crack use. Police officers say that fighting crack is like fighting a war. They say it is a war they are losing.

The Cocaine Road

It's a long road from the mountains of South America to the streets of the United States. It's the cocaine road.

The cocaine road begins in the mountain villages of Peru, Bolivia, and Colombia. Here, South American farmers, most of them very poor, grow and tend the coca plants. For many of these farmers, growing coca is the way they make enough money to feed and clothe their families. Over 400,000 acres of South American farmland are now used to grow the coca plant.

The road travels from these poor mountain villages to small cocaine laboratories hidden deep in the South American jungle. The farmer sells his coca leaves to a "mule," a man who turns the leaves into coca paste. The coca leaves are first dried in the sun; then, they are soaked in strong chemicals such as sulfuric acid and gasoline to make a coca paste. The mule carries this paste to small jungle labs. Here, even more chemicals are used to turn the paste into cocaine powder. Now, the drug is ready for sale in the United States.

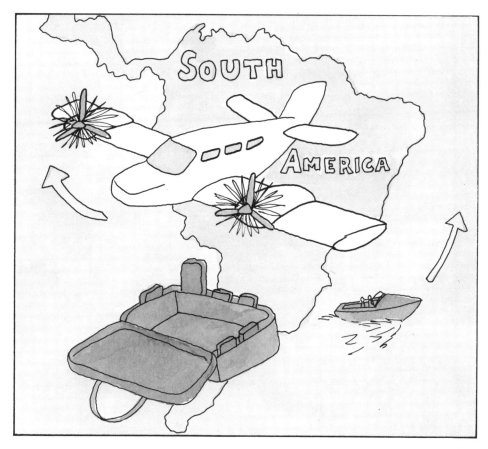

The road travels by sea and air from South America to the United States. Drug smugglers sneak cocaine into this country. They hide big drug shipments on planes and boats. They place smaller shipments in packages and suitcases. They even tape packets of cocaine to their bodies. Over 400 tons of cocaine are smuggled out of South America each year. Half of this cocaine comes to the United States.

The road travels to "safe houses" in cities across America. Here, the drug shipment is held until a dealer is ready to pick it up. The drug dealer, also called a pusher, is the person who sells the drug to cocaine users. In order to make more money, dealers "cut" the cocaine by adding cheap fillers, like flour and baking soda, or less expensive drugs. The drug they sell as "cocaine" may be only 10% to 75% pure cocaine.

Every stop on the cocaine road is controlled by drug criminals. In South America, large drug gangs use bribes and violence to keep the drug road open. In the United States, dealers set up drug rings and hire people, sometimes young people, to sell cocaine. The cocaine business is a big one—over $100 billion a year.

Can the drug road be shut down? Many people are trying to do just that. Soldiers and drug enforcement officials attack the jungle labs in South America. Police in the United States raid "rock houses," where crack is made and sold.

But it is not enough. The drug trade is too big. It will take more than police and soldiers to shut down the cocaine road. One police officer from Los Angeles said the same thing: "The answer has to be something else."

Cocaine and the Body

Len Bias was a star on the basketball court. He was in perfect health. But cocaine killed Len Bias. He was only 22 years old when he died.

Leonard Bias played basketball for the University of Maryland. He was no average player, however. Many people said he was the best college basketball player in the country. The Boston Celtics thought so. Two days before his death, he was drafted No. 1 by the Celtics to play professional basketball. "He could jump through the roof," said Red Auerbach, the president of the Celtics.

Len Bias snorted cocaine the night of his death. It may have been the first time he ever used the drug. It was certainly the last time. Cocaine stopped his heart.

The news of Len Bias's death sent thousands of callers to cocaine hotlines across the country. "How could such a star athlete be killed by cocaine?" they wanted to know. "Could it happen to me? How much cocaine is safe to use?"

The answer is simple. "No amount of cocaine is safe," says Dr. Jeffrey Eisner of the New England Medical Center Hospitals. Using coke only once can cause serious damage to the body. Dr. Louis Caplan, also from the New England Medical Center Hospitals, says that using cocaine is like taking a chance on sudden death: "Cocaine's a loaded gun."

How could cocaine kill a young, healthy athlete?

To understand this, let's take a look at what cocaine does to the body.

Your body is a wonderful system of many different parts. The parts of your body—like the brain, or the heart, or the lungs—have important jobs to do. They all work together to keep you alive and healthy. But it's your job to keep them healthy, too. Using cocaine makes your body sick.

Here are some of the ways cocaine can damage the human body:

• The Brain

Your brain is the control center of your body. It sends out and receives billions and billions of electrical signals every day. These messages speed along from one nerve cell (called a neuron) to the next until they reach every part of your body. The signals from the brain control the heart and lungs and the other parts of your body. They direct your movements, thoughts, and feelings.

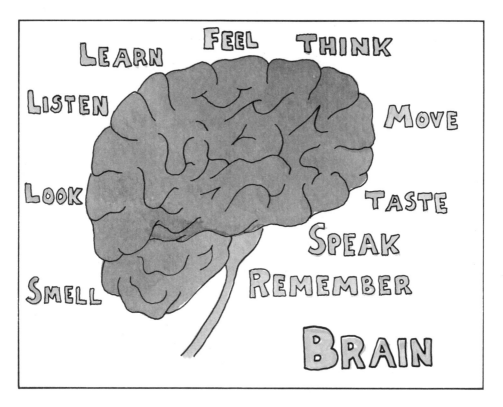

But cocaine is a stimulant. It speeds up the way the brain works. When cocaine is used, the brain may send out too many electrical signals. This can lead to a seizure. A seizure means that the brain's electrical messages get all mixed-up. It causes the mind to go blank. It may cause the body to shake all over and become stiff. Using cocaine can lead to a series of these seizures—and damage to the brain. Cocaine can also cause the blood vessels of the brain to burst. This is called a "stroke," and it can lead to brain damage—and sudden death.

• The Heart

The heart is a muscle about the size and shape of your fist. It pumps blood to every part of the body. Day and night, the heart keeps pumping and pumping in a regular rhythm— more than 100,000 times a day. Inside the heart is a special area called the pacemaker. The pacemaker keeps the heart pumping by sending out little electrical signals that tell the heart muscles to beat. The pacemaker is controlled by the brain. Messages from the brain tell the pacemaker to speed up or slow down.

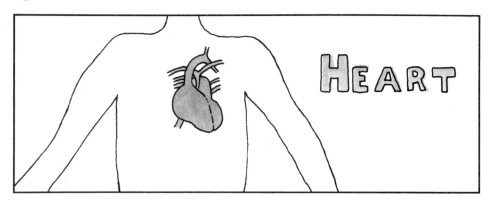

But cocaine makes the heart pump too fast. The messages from the brain that control the pacemaker make the heart beat so fast that the muscles of the heart may be damaged. It can also disrupt the electrical signals from the pacemaker that keep the heart pumping. Using cocaine could lead to a sudden heart attack—and sudden death.

• The Lungs

Our lungs breathe in the air we need to live, and breathe out the air our bodies no longer need. Take a deep breath. Hold it. Did you feel your lungs fill up with air? Breathing in is how the body gets the oxygen it needs to live. The oxygen enters the bloodstream, and the heart pumps it throughout the body. Like the other parts of your body, the lungs are controlled by the brain. A special control area in the brain sends out electrical signals that tell the lungs how fast and how deep to breathe. Now, let that breath out. Phew!

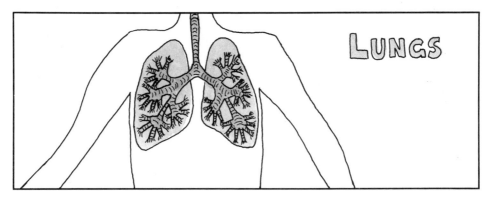

But using cocaine hurts the lungs. Smoking cocaine leads to shortness of breath and makes it harder for the lungs to get oxygen into the blood. Using cocaine in any way can also stop the brain from sending out those electrical signals that keep the lungs breathing. That will cause the lungs to stop working—and sudden death.

Cocaine Babies

The baby shook and jittered in the hospital nursery. His mother was young and frightened.

"What's the matter with my baby?" she asked the nurse on duty.

The nurse explained that the newborn infant was showing the signs of cocaine withdrawal.

"Cocaine?" was the mother's startled response. She didn't know that using coke would hurt her baby.

"Cocaine," said the nurse.

"It's a new problem, but a very real one," says one doctor. The problem is cocaine babies—babies born to mothers who used cocaine while they were pregnant. If women use coke during the time they are pregnant, there is a good chance their children will be drug damaged, too.

Like other drugs, cocaine is passed from the pregnant mother to her unborn baby. As bad as cocaine is for an adult, it is even worse for a baby.

Cocaine babies are often born too early. They are smaller and lighter than other babies. Their bodies are not fully formed, and they may develop lung diseases or brain damage.

Cocaine babies are shaky and tense, and they may go into spasms when they are touched. They may be very irritable. They have trouble paying attention to the world around them. Dr. Ira Chasnoff, who works with cocaine babies at Northwestern Memorial Hospital in Chicago, says, "These babies can't focus on a human face or respond to a human voice."

Many of the mothers of cocaine babies are poor. Often, they are addicted to crack. But it's not just poor women who are having cocaine babies. Many people, rich as well as poor, do not realize that using coke will hurt their unborn babies. And some women who use cocaine or crack may not know that they are, in fact, pregnant.

Thousands of cocaine babies are born each year. It may take many months and even years for cocaine babies to get well. Some may never fully get over the damage to their young bodies. Many doctors think that cocaine babies will have more problems when they go to school. They may have trouble with language and learning skills; they may have behavior problems. As one doctor said, "We are only now beginning to realize how serious this could be."

These are just some of the problems caused by cocaine use. Cocaine users may also suffer from dizziness, coughing, sinus headaches, and sore throats. They may not be able to eat or sleep well. They may have tremors, headaches, vomiting, nosebleeds, muscle pains, and many other problems.

Coke users often mix cocaine with other drugs. This combination of drugs is even more dangerous to the body than using cocaine by itself. And people who use needles to inject cocaine also run the risk of getting serious diseases like hepatitis and AIDS.

Len Bias probably did not know how dangerous cocaine is. Or maybe he thought it wouldn't hurt him. But it did. Reverend Jesse Jackson spoke at Len Bias's funeral. He spoke about the lesson of his death, the lesson of cocaine. "On a day the children mourn," Reverend Jackson said, "I hope they learn."

Red Auerbach gave Len Bias's team jersey, No. 30, to the Bias family. It had never been worn.

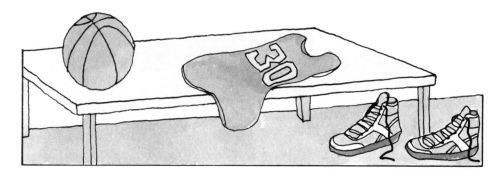

Cocaine and Addiction

It may seem like fun, just something to try. It may be something new to do at a party or with a group of friends. But using cocaine doesn't stay fun for long.

Because the cocaine high lasts for such a short time, people who use cocaine often use it over and over again. They find that they need more and more cocaine to feel the drug's effects. They need more cocaine just *not* to feel bad. They are addicted to cocaine. Dr. Ron Siegel, who studies cocaine at the University of California at Los Angeles, says it is easier to get hooked on coke than any other drug.

How easy is it to get hooked on cocaine? Many users say they felt hooked the very first time they tried it. One woman, after trying coke for the first time, said it took only "30 seconds" for her to become dependent on coke. One man, after his first try, said, "I swear, in two hours I was on my way to becoming an addict."

What is it like to be addicted to cocaine? Scientists have studied cocaine addiction in monkeys and rats. This is what they learned in their experiments:

- When offered the choice of food or cocaine, rats chose coke. They would rather starve than give up cocaine.

- Rats chose cocaine even if that meant they were given electrical shocks. They would rather feel painful jolts of electricity than give up cocaine.

- Monkeys will keep giving themselves doses of cocaine until they die. They would rather die than give up cocaine.

- In order to get a single dose of cocaine, monkeys will perform the same task (like pressing a special bar) over 12,800 times. They would rather do anything than give up cocaine.

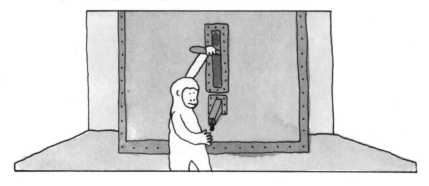

But monkeys and rats don't show us what being addicted to cocaine is really like. Here is the picture of a coke habit:

- Addiction is a 19-year-old woman who sells her jewelry to get money for coke. But, soon, she is broke again. She starts selling crack on the street.

- Addiction is a 24-year-old major league baseball player who is caught using cocaine. He has one more chance to give up coke. But he can't. He gets caught again and is kicked out of baseball for life.

- Addiction is a 27-year-old mother of three who spends all of her money on drugs. She leaves her children at home alone while she looks for another dose of cocaine.

- Addiction is a 41-year-old man who doesn't care if he loses his business or if his family leaves him. "Nothing comes before my cocaine," he says.

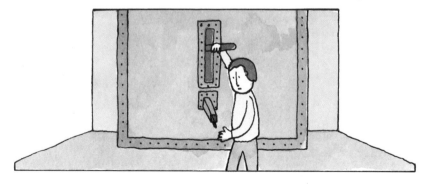

Cocaine changes the moods and feelings of the people who use it. They may become nervous and easily upset. They may feel that people are "out to get them." They may get depressed and even think about committing suicide.

Coke users often see or hear things that aren't really there. These are called hallucinations. Some coke users say they feel insects crawling under the skin—this hallucination is known as "coke bugs" or "snow bugs."

Nothing is more important to coke addicts than cocaine. They lose interest in everything else: how they look, whether or not they eat, how sick coke makes them, what they are doing to their family and friends. They will lie or cheat or steal to get another dose of cocaine. Often, they sell drugs to make enough money to buy more cocaine.

Two out of every three callers to the 800-COCAINE hotline said they were unable to stop using coke despite trying to again and again. Why can't they just stop using the drug?

That is a difficult question to answer. Scientists are now trying to find the answer by studying what cocaine does to the brain. We have seen that the brain controls our moods and feelings. It makes us feel good or bad. It seems that cocaine helps to release the kinds of chemicals that make us feel good. But it may be that the brain of the coke user stops releasing these chemicals by itself. It depends on the cocaine to do that. So the coke user now needs the drug to feel good.

One thing we know for sure: users who try to stop taking coke feel terrible. They feel upset, depressed, nervous, tired, and sick. But most of all, they feel a very strong need for more cocaine. These sick feelings are part of what is called cocaine withdrawal. Coke addicts get so used to the drug that they need more cocaine just to feel normal.

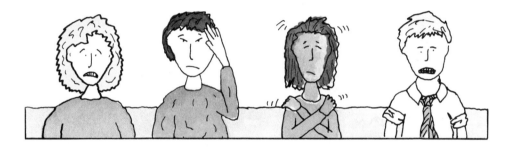

Then, is there any help for people hooked on cocaine?

Yes, it is possible for cocaine users to get over their drug addiction. But it is not easy. The road to cocaine addiction is like a fast and furious roller coaster ride. But the road back is like a long and hard climb up a steep mountain.

People who are hooked on cocaine need help. They can't break the coke habit by themselves. Many coke users refuse to believe they have a drug problem at all. This is called denial. The families of coke users need help, too. It is hard to admit that a family member has a drug problem. We may even try to cover up a drug problem by making excuses or just by looking the other way. This is called enabling.

Statements of Denial

People who use cocaine often refuse to believe they have a drug problem. This is called denial. Here are some ways people deny a drug problem:

"I only use coke on the weekend. It's no big deal."

"I'm not hurting anyone, am I?"

"I like to party. Is there anything wrong with that?"

"I can stop whenever I feel like it."

"It's my money. I can spend it the way I want."

Statements of Enabling

It is hard to admit that a person we know has a drug problem. Sometimes, we look the other way, or we just don't do anything at all. This is called enabling. Here are some ways people enable a drug problem:

"It's not hurting his schoolwork."

"It's just a stage she's going through."

"What should we do? Call the police on our child?"

"Let's wait another week and see what happens."

"What can we do about it?"

It doesn't help to deny or enable a drug problem. The only way to stop cocaine use is to face the problem head-on: to learn the truth about cocaine and to get treatment. There are places coke users can turn to for help. There are people who will help coke users live a drug-free life.

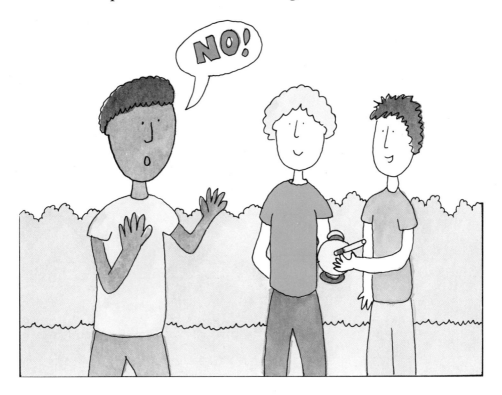

There is one other way to stop cocaine use. It's the best way. It's simple, easy, and safe.

What is it?

The best way to stop cocaine is never to start.

Cocaine: The Big Lie

"I was just lying to myself," one coke user said over and over to herself. "Lie after lie after lie."

The National Institute on Drug Abuse calls cocaine and crack "The Big Lie." That's because there are many wrong ideas about the drug. Here are some of those wrong ideas and the facts about cocaine:

"Cocaine powder is for the rich. Crack is for the poor."

That's a lie. It used to be that cocaine powder was very expensive, but it is not anymore. Now, it is cheap enough for most people to afford. Studies show no difference in the amount of cocaine powder used in rich and poor areas. It used to be that crack was found only in the poor areas of major cities, but not anymore. Now, it is used in wealthy suburbs and small towns. Crack is used by people of all races, by men and women, by old people and young.

"Using coke only once can't hurt you."

That's a lie. Using coke only once can kill you. One dose of cocaine can disrupt the electrical signals from the brain to the heart and lungs. They may suddenly stop working—and that means death. One dose of cocaine can cause a stroke. That's when blood vessels in the brain burst—and that can mean permanent damage to the brain.

"It's safe to sniff cocaine."

That's a lie. Some people think you won't get addicted to cocaine if you only sniff it, but that's a lie, too. A study of the phone calls to 800-COCAINE, the national cocaine hotline, showed that many of the people who needed help with cocaine problems only sniffed the drug. Sniffing cocaine can lead to serious damage to the lining of the nose, the sinuses, and throughout the respiratory system. It, too, can mean a chance for sudden death.

The End of the Story

There are signs that people are starting to get the message about cocaine. A recent survey of high-school seniors by the National Institute on Drug Abuse shows that cocaine use is down for the second year in a row.

That's a good sign. But it doesn't mean the cocaine story will have a happy ending. The cocaine story is not over yet.

On July 5, 1989, two U.S. Coast Guard ships stopped a freighter from the Central American country of Panama. The freighter was carrying cement to the United States. But hidden deep in the ship was a roomful of cocaine. It was one of the largest cocaine seizures of 1989—3,359 pounds of cocaine.

That should be good news, too. After all, 3,359 pounds is a lot of cocaine.

But even that much is not enough to stop the illegal flow of cocaine. It is not even close. Coke users in the United States sniff, inject, or smoke that much cocaine every week.

What *will* stop the coke habit?

The police, the courts, the Coast Guard—they will stop some of it. But they are not the whole answer.

The answer lies with you. What happens in the future is up to you and thousands of boys and girls like you.

It's up to you to decide that you can have fun without drugs.

It's up to you to decide that you can solve your problems without drugs.

It's up to you to know the truth about cocaine—and to act on what you know.

This book has given you the facts about cocaine. Now, it's up to you to say "No" to coke and end the cocaine story once and for all.

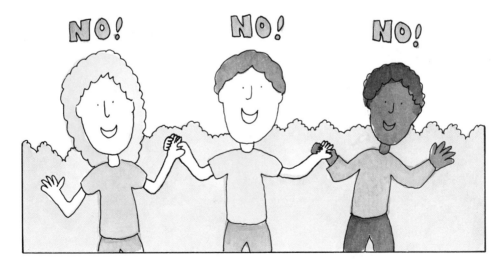

GLOSSARY

addiction	the constant need or craving that makes people use drugs they know are harmful
coca	the plant from which cocaine comes
cocaine	a drug that comes from the leaves of the coca plant
coke	another word for cocaine
coke bugs	the hallucination that insects are crawling under the skin; also called snow bugs
crack	a form of cocaine that is made to be smoked
crash	the sick feeling cocaine users get when the effects of the drug wear off
dealer	a person who sells illegal drugs; another word for pusher
denial	when a person refuses to believe that a drug problem exists
dependence	the way the body and brain need a drug to avoid feeling sick
drug	a substance that changes the way the brain works

enabling	when the family or friends of drug users overlook drug-related problems
euphoria	a feeling of great happiness and pleasure
gateway drug	a drug that can lead to other drug problems
hallucination	a false or mistaken idea sometimes caused by drug use
mule	a person who transports coca leaves to cocaine laboratories
peer pressure	the feeling that you have to do something because other people your age are doing it
pusher	another word for dealer
rock houses	houses where crack is made and sold; also called crack houses
smuggler	a person who sneaks illegal drugs into a country
stimulant	a kind of drug that speeds up the way the brain works
tolerance	the way the body and brain need more and more of a drug to get the same effect
withdrawal	the sick feeling drug users get when they can't get the drugs they are dependent on

Index